The Dog
Always Cooks

The Dog Always Cooks

DEBORAH ROBBINS-GILES

StoryTerrace

Text StoryTerrace

Design StoryTerrace and Jelena Žarko

Copyright © Deborah Robbins-Giles

First print April 2022

StoryTerrace

www.StoryTerrace.com

CONTENTS

FOREWORD

irstly, I would like to thank everyone who encouraged me to write this book; especially, my husband Paul. I would also like to thank my friends, and friends of my father for letting me 'bend their ear' over the years. The past decade and a half has been one hell of a ride. When you decide to look after elderly people, it is not to be taken lightly because it will test your relationship to the max. As time progresses, should the elderly people develop dementia, you will have no time for yourself at all and will probably, like me, end up even having to cut that person's food up to feed them. There will be highs and lows along the way. I truly believe that you come out the other end a far stronger person, you will do things that you never could have seen yourself doing, and you learn so much about yourself. I have written this book in a way that hopefully will give you, the reader, a true perspective of what is involved day to day. I have also included some useful tips that I picked up along the way, which I wish I had known at the start …

1

STICKING TOGETHER DEFINES A FAMILY

Our dogs are the centre of our universe. Paul and I live for them, our beautiful labradoodles who share the home we have lived in for 21 years. They heal us in our recovery, our recovery from the lockdown that has exhausted and drained us for a decade and a half, but the life which we would choose all over again, without a shadow of a doubt.

I want to write this book to share the lifestyle we chose to live, the way of life that some friends, colleagues and family members questioned, 'Why?' 'How?' Nobody seems to think they would want nor have the energy to choose what we chose. Let me take you on my journey from the day it all began when our lives were voluntarily put on hold as my husband, Paul, and I revolved our lives around Auntie Rita and my dad. My hope is that our experiences will help and guide others as they consider the possibility of caring for their aged, loved ones themselves.

I had lost my mum when she was just 62. She had suffered for five years from cancer, and I suppose I had lots of space left to love others in my grieving heart. Dad was five years older than Mum.

About three years after moving into our new home I was working as usual, receiving calls at the ambulance service, when a call came in with an address I recognised. My auntie Rita, Dad's sister, had fallen and hurt her arm. There had been a stage of life where none of us had been in regular contact with Auntie Rita – there had been a few family misunderstandings.

However, Dad had bumped into his sister, Rita, at the local library and, as was his forgiving nature, he had immediately let bygones be bygones when he saw her and remembered how close they had been and the good old days. He had suggested that she moved in with them when Mum was still alive and Mum had agreed to this. I loved my dad completely and I'd do anything he asked. Therefore, when he wondered if I could look after his sister as her arm injury had made her unable to care for herself, I had no reservation. I made the solemn promise to my dad that I would look after his sister for him, in our home, until her dying day.

Auntie had lived in a lovely bungalow in Sedgley where she had employed a gardener. She hated cooking and lived off sandwiches and ready meals from Marks and Spencer. She had her own car, but she was becoming too elderly to drive and didn't particularly enjoy it anymore.

Prim and proper Auntie Rita was soon settled into her new home with us. She happily sold all her furniture but asked to bring her grandfather clock. She also brought lots of keepsakes that she had inherited from her parents and grandparents, and they are still in storage. She used to like watching, 'Dickinson's Real Deal,' and wanted us to start a business selling her things. Unfortunately, she'd have an idea like this, but it would dissolve into nothing and the next day she would have no interest. So, her family heirlooms stayed in storage and we used to joke with her that whenever we admired an item on the show that we probably had a copy.

I quickly learnt to respond to her summons as she clicked her fingers at me. We all had to adapt to our new life together and I had to swallow a huge dose of empathy and understanding in order to view life from the same perspective as my darling spinster aunt with her high expectations.

I am naturally a caring and affectionate person and I love to fuss over things and look after people. Dad said that as a child I was always very sensitive and affectionate, and I would gladly share my sweets, toys and pocket money. I soon grew fond of Auntie Rita with her high and mighty idiosyncrasies and over the years this developed into love.

Having no siblings, I was always very close to my parents, and we had all thoroughly enjoyed family life, the three of us going everywhere together. My childhood comes with nothing but happy memories. We lived near Sedgley Beacon at the time, where Dad would take me tobogganing with his homemade sledge and we'd sit on it together. I had every confidence in him as he worked the brakes. Dad took me on camping adventures, and we would regularly go to the swimming pool or for our long walks. Even when I was seventeen years old, he'd take me and a friend camping with his friends, ensuring that any strangers we encountered knew that I was his daughter! Looking back, Dad was very patient with us especially when it came to getting ready – we had to do make-up before we went on the daily adventure and that certainly took some time! When I was five, he gave in to my pestering to accompany him on his long drive for a business appointment in Hereford. He was such a good soul because once we got there, and I'd had something to eat, I announced I was bored so he drove me all the way home and had to rearrange his meeting! When Dad and I were on our rambles Mum would wait contentedly in the car and read. The extended family were always involved in our lives, and it was my grandad (Mum's dad) who taught me to read even before I started school. Some days the teacher would even have me stand up and read a book or the paper to the class! Both my parents were excellent at parenting and ensured that I was never a spoilt only child! My grandmother lived with my parents in her final few years, and only died when I was 28. I saw how my mum cared for her so well and I guess she was a role model for what I was to undertake later.

When I was in a school play as Brer rabbit Grandma made my outfit. I was raised in a generation where parents used smacking as a form of discipline. Dad only ever smacked me twice. Once when I was five, I kicked my mum because she wouldn't give me my own way on a matter! When I was eleven, I was rude to my gran. After those times Dad just needed to give me, 'the look'. As I loved my parents, I tried to behave anyway.

When Auntie Rita joined Dad in coming to live with us, we started going everywhere together, it was like recreating the times from when I was younger. To say that there was a massive change to our lifestyle is an understatement. I didn't like some of the changes and I knew I couldn't alter them, so I had to change my approach. Some people said that I must be very placid but to tell the truth, I soon came to realise acceptance was better than anger and if I couldn't change things, I could change my mindset. One of the huge changes I didn't like was the huge increase in washing. Having an empty laundry basket was the best one second of the month!

Dad was happy to eat whatever we were eating but Auntie Rita was a monkey, well actually a bit of a devil! Her persona gave off vibes that she was starring as a lady from the series, 'Upstairs, Downstairs', and I was one of the maids! As I placed her meal on the table, she would demand, 'What's this? This isn't what I want to eat today.'

At first, I would say, 'Come on, I'm at work. You know I

THE DOG ALWAYS COOKS

can't prepare different meals.' I soon learnt that she would always have a strong comeback, which indicated that she clearly only saw things from her perspective: 'Yes but I've come to live here now and you wait on me.' Even when Auntie's mental condition deteriorated there was no bluffing her! I couldn't serve fish if she wanted chicken; she was a lady who always got what she wanted and life was easier that way!

In the early days I decided to take Auntie Rita on a shopping trip – after all a bit of retail therapy is known for bonding women's friendships – but I made the huge mistake of taking her to Birmingham market for clothes!

'What's this?' the curt shrill voice cut the air and all the traders seemed to turn and stare as they heard her. 'I like names,' she continued. 'Oh no I don't like this,' her loud voice seemed to stand out above the general buzz of the market hustle and bustle. She was like a naughty, petulant toddler who wanted her favourite toyshop, so to keep the peace I took her to her favourite department store where her face lit up as she saw all the designer brands. She wouldn't wear any shoes apart from Clark's shoes.

Auntie had been a manager at the Midland Electricity Board, and she had clearly been exceptionally good at her job as I automatically found myself respecting her authority in every area of life. Clear, concise instructions just flew out of her mouth with such confidence and self-belief that they would be followed to the letter. I found it easier to conform to her wishes rather than try to change the mind that I soon realised had never seen life from another person's point of view.

Dad explained that she had always had high expectations in life and had never married because no man had ever met these high standards which she set. She'd been on the search for a Rock Hudson lookalike, who was a doctor or barrister, to marry but sadly never found one who returned her attention. She had always lived a high-class lifestyle, loving her hobbies of horse riding and tennis and apparently, she holidayed abroad in the days before the general population did. Dad said that as her friends married, their lives took them on a different path, and one by one, they drifted away from her. Auntie Rita and Dad, as I was led to believe, were descendants of the family who made the anchor for the ill-fated Titanic. Sometimes during the following years, I felt I had been shipwrecked and could have done with a good anchor!

I soon learnt that Aunt saw me as her servant and it was made very clear that she had no intention of doing jobs around the house! Auntie was sat reading a book on one of her first mornings with us and I was dashing around like a headless chicken, tidying up before I left for work. I suggested that she might like to flick a duster around because I wouldn't be home until late afternoon. I should have known better as the self-assured voice told me in no uncertain tones, 'I've not come here to do work. I've come here for you to do the work. I'm just reading this book.'

We soon came to know our new family member had a very strong mind of her own and stubborn was her middle name! We had made the commitment to look after her and I had promised my dad that I would. Sometimes people don't understand the promises they are making when they agree to them, and I hadn't comprehended the obstinate nature of our new lodger. I loved my dad so much that I knew I would never break my promise to him even if the promise threatened to break me. Thankfully, I soon realised that my growing love for my aunt was like a river, always changing with the weather and seasons of her moods and actions but it continued to flow – even though on some days it was just a trickle!

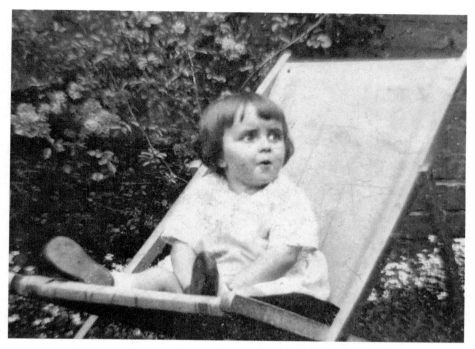

Auntie Rita taking in the fresh air in the 1920s.

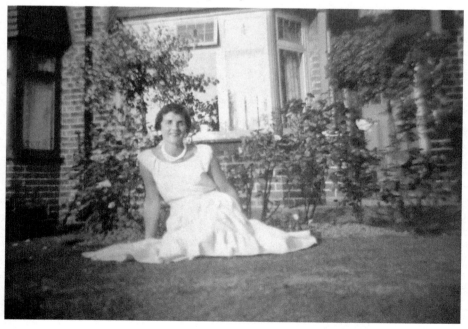

Auntie Rita dressed beautifully in her 20s.

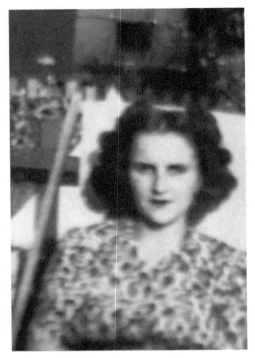

Very glam Auntie Rita in the 1940s.

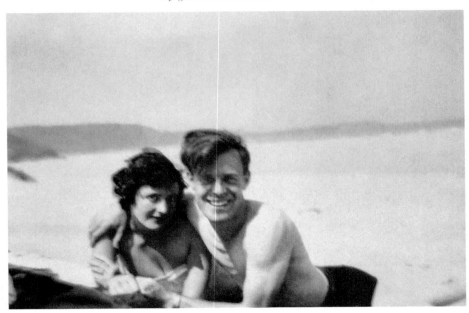

Mum and Dad on their honeymoon in Cornwall in 1957.

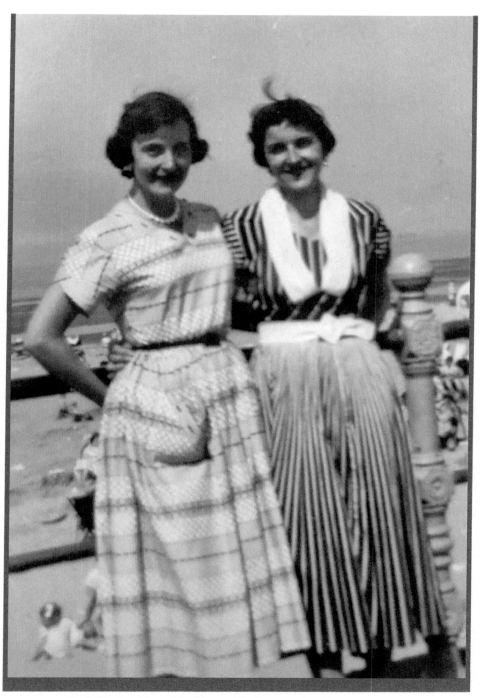

Auntie Rita and Mum whilst Mum and Dad were courting. Taken in the 1950s.

2

THE LIGHTS START TO FLICKER

Dad was happy having his big sister with him permanently and Auntie Rita had apparently had her dream come true. Dad revealed that she had always assumed that her and Dad would live together before my mother had come onto the scene. Apparently, Auntie Rita had loved the old television series, 'Sykes and A...' where Eric Sykes and Hattie Jacques played twins living together at 24 Sebastopol Terrace. The theme of each episode completed the title. She had earmarked Dad to do all the cooking, driving and DIY, etc. Dad explained that his sister had always been rather spoilt and that she was now treating me as she had their mother! She would throw items of her clothing at me and command, 'You can wash that again. I've come to live here as a guest.' She had obviously taken very literally Dad's words that if she came to live with us I would do absolutely everything and care for her completely. After all, this was the promise, I had given my dad. He recalled that as children she would bully him and twist his wrist around until he met her demands but one day, when he was about thirteen, he had given her a taste of her own medicine and she stopped it all then.

Auntie loved the bedroom we provided for her with her four-poster bed with its pink drapes and the television at the bottom of the bed. Dad's health was failing so I tried my best to prepare healthy meals and provide regular exercise for Dad and his sister. Thankfully, we all had a hobby in common – we loved walking. One weekend morning I decided to lead us all on a ramble near Worcester which I had found in a local newspaper. We were all kitted out in hiking boots, and I was relaxing in the beautiful scenery when I noticed Dad slowing down and looking rather off-colour. From what I had learnt from working for the Ambulance Service, alarm bells started to go off in my head. Dad was portraying all the classic signs of a heart attack, but we were literally in a field in the middle of nowhere! In those days, reception, on our brick of a mobile, was poor so Paul was sent to get help! Auntie Rita was running round in circles, screaming, 'He's going to die,' which of course, were not the words her brother needed to hear just then! Dad had turned a very nasty colour. Paul scrambled across pastures to a house we'd seen on the distant horizon, and he was lucky to catch the family as they were piling into their car. By good fortune, the daughter had just passed her final medic exams, so Dad was soon in good hands as we awaited the ambulance which they kindly had phoned for, from their house. They had even carried a chair for Dad across all the fields. Of course, Auntie Rita was eyeing the chair up for herself!

It was discovered that Dad had suffered previous heart attacks and his heart was badly damaged. I immediately started to research more suitable diets for him and I often ended up having to prepare a completely different dish for our new epicure! Auntie still wouldn't help by agreeing to eat the same meals. The hospital told us that Dad's heart attack was severe and there was insufficient muscle left to benefit from a bypass operation. The only treatment was medication. We were shocked to be given a prognosis of just six years. I dedicated myself even more to waiting on him hand and foot and thankfully he lived for a further fourteen years.

While Dad was still in the hospital, we'd ask his sister if she was coming to visit. She revealed spoilt, childish behaviour in so many ways and if an activity wasn't centred around her, she would play up no end. We weren't comfortable leaving her home alone so bribery was sometimes used to get her into the car to visit Dad. Likewise, she'd only agree to accompany me to the supermarket if I promised to buy her whichever treats she fancied.

Not long after this episode, I walked into the beautiful bedroom that we had furnished for Auntie Rita like a suite from a five-star hotel. The deep pile rose-pink luxury carpet had cost a small fortune, but we wanted Auntie to continue living the lifestyle she had developed for herself in her own home. 'What do you think you're doing?' my amazed lips probably thundered as the '£' signs from the carpet bill were still fresh in my mind.

Auntie Rita had decided to relieve herself and deposit the contents of her bowels on this new carpet! Goodness knows how but I managed to calm my immediate reaction and kindly say, 'Come on let's get you cleaned up.' I gently led her to the bathroom and ensured she was clean and comfortable, in a new set of clothes, before I took her downstairs to watch one of her favourite colourful videos. Paul wondered why he found me on my hands and knees scrubbing the new carpet and I let Auntie maintain her dignity as I mumbled,

'Auntie Rita had a tiny accident and spilt something on the carpet.'

That was the first day I think I earnt my halo which later some friends joked that they could see. It was also the first day that I fully understood that life was going to change even more with many such steep learning curves for Paul and me to face. The realisation hit me that sadly, Auntie Rita was displaying signs of dementia.

Paul and I realised we would have to introduce a strict bathing schedule, and it made obvious sense that I would take responsibility for the personal hygiene tasks with Aunt, and Paul would look after Dad's bathroom requirements. I kept the medication for Dad and Auntie's heart problems locked safely away in my bedroom upstairs, and I had a routine time each day to administer it. I used to fully moisturise

Auntie and Dad each day to keep their skin lovely and soft!

I would set the table in the dining room each day and cook a three-course meal for Dad and Auntie Rita as I went to work, leaving sandwiches for their evening meal. Dad would patiently sit and prompt his sister to eat. I went to the seminars at the local hospital to discover recipe and meal suggestions that would cater best for each of their conditions. Auntie would attend the sessions with me as I tried to discover ways to promote their good health through nutrition.

We had leather sofas but kept covers on them which were washed daily as were all the bedsheets. Auntie Rita could be like Goldilocks trying out all the beds in one night, regardless of the fact somebody else might be in them. When she climbed in with Paul and me, she would fidget so much that Paul would go and sleep on the sofa downstairs while she continued to sleep beside me. We bought a huge tumble dryer which was on non-stop. When I used to take Auntie to the doctors, and I'd see old people in the waiting room with partners who were obviously ill I used to think I don't know how old people look after old people. I knew from my experiences the levels of energy needed. I was on duty eighteen hours per day and sleep was always interrupted. I used to take Auntie and Dad to their personal appointments, and I was totally embarrassed when she decided to tell a man to let me have a seat in the waiting room because I was 'knackered.'

Dad had always loved swimming and I felt this activity would be beneficial to both Dad's and Auntie Rita's health. So, Paul and I bought subscriptions for us all at the local private spa and leisure centre. We all soon became regulars, attending about three or four times a week. Unfortunately, Auntie couldn't swim although she loved sitting by the poolside looking at a newspaper, even though she often had it upside down! As her illness further stole her abilities, the team at the leisure centre showed great patience and assistance by helping us with her less sociable habits.

As the dementia progressed, I enjoyed some backhanded compliments from Auntie: 'I don't know who she is,' she'd point at me, 'but she's very good at housekeeping.'

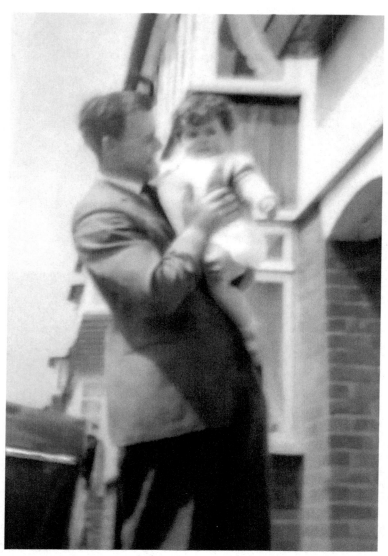

My proud Dad and I in 1962.

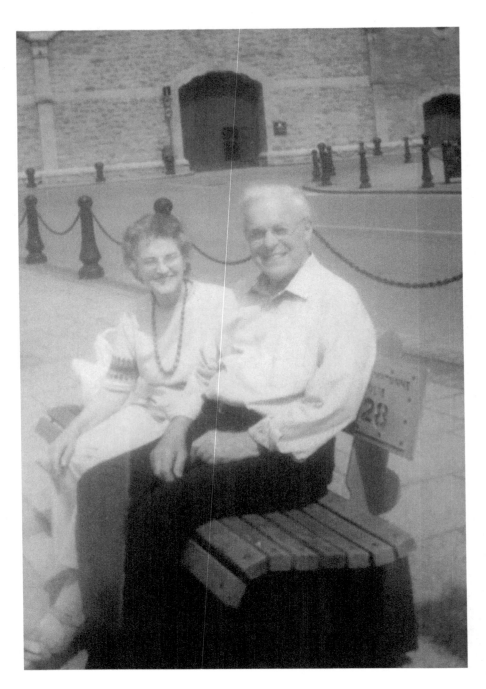

Dad and Auntie Rita in Jersey in the mid 1990s.

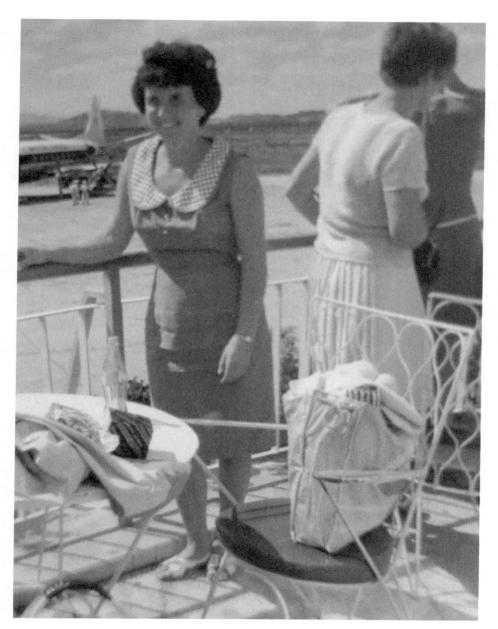

Auntie Rita at the airport, circa 1960.

3

TO LOVE A PERSON IS
TO LEARN THE SONG
THAT IS IN THEIR HEART

Paul, Dad and I tried to learn the song in Auntie Rita's heart and to sing it to her when she had forgotten. By that I mean that we all tried to find ways of helping Auntie to have the best quality of life possible by incorporating into her daily life things we knew she liked. None of us let our frustrations show when she couldn't remember, and we didn't try to make her understand. We tried to let her know of our love by just being her companion, sometimes, if she allowed, we'd sit and hold her hand. We reminded ourselves daily that her confusion meant that her sometimes cruel or socially unacceptable words and phrases were not meant.

Auntie would talk about the royal family, an interest of hers, so we would read up about the ones she thought were still alive. She particularly liked Queen Victoria and the Victorian Era and some days she believed that we were living in that era. We learnt to research more into her hobbies. When I was a child Dad used to dance with me; he taught me the foxtrot and the waltz. My grandma had taught me the Charleston. So, I tried to recreate our family dance sessions which had been great fun. I even sent off for some 1920s and 1940s dance costumes for us all to wear as I recreated that era. What splendid afternoon tea dances we all had. Dad used to say, 'You're zany our Debs!' Auntie Rita loved to dance and once we took her to a family celebration where there was a proper disco floor with flashing lights. We couldn't get Auntie Rita off the dance floor as she showed off all her moves. She always picked out the handsome men to dance with – no fool! My sister-in-law's husband particularly took her fancy as she stalked him around the dancefloor! At the cinema showing of, 'Mamma Mia!' – my friend, who had gone with us, was mortified when Auntie Rita got up and wouldn't stop dancing in the aisles to each song. One early evening, we were walking with our oldest dog (only had the one then) in Worcester when we passed a nightclub where the lady who was opening up caught sight of him. She made a huge fuss over him and, clearly a dog lover, she invited us into the nightclub. Once inside, Auntie spotted the dancefloor. Disco fever took her straight into her dance moves! She was like a child in a chocolate factory. We were all so busy watching all her incredible steps that we didn't notice the dog helping himself to the remnants of a discarded vodka! We had to keep an eye out for him that night!

I still ensured that I took library books out that Auntie

had loved before this cruel illness took hold. Dad had a library card and loved to choose a selection of books so we'd all go on a family trip to the library. Auntie had told me how she enjoyed reading biographies and the classics like Jane Eyre. I would now find time to read her passages in the hope of relieving her agitated and confused mind. She enjoyed audible books and seemed to like hearing Alan Titchmarsh; for some reason, his voice calmed her. She had loved watching Columbo on television and we found that she'd be happy to sit still for longer, in her favourite armchair, if we played some of her old favourites. The familiar theme tunes and voices she recognised seemed to appease her troubled mind. We soon discovered the bright shows that featured dancing and music and beautiful costumes still managed to hold some of her interests.

I often felt particularly sad for Dad when his sister would ask him if he was ready for school. He'd calmly reply, I'm not going today. You get ready though.' If she'd died, he'd have missed her, if she'd moved area, he'd have missed her but here she was living with him and he still missed the real Auntie Rita every day. It was obviously distressing for Dad when she asked where their parents were and it seemed to be cruel to tell her each time that they had passed away and to watch the grief strike her yet again. It was much kinder to pretend they were in the other room or that they weren't home yet.

We learnt to banish background noises when we wanted

to converse with Auntie and to keep to short sentences. Arguments were a big no-no and none of us were really the argumentative type anyway. Routine became important to try and regulate some sort of body clock for Auntie. I bought caffeine-free tea and coffee to try to ensure that we did everything to get us all a few extra minutes of sleep at night. We tried to limit daytime naps for the same reason. Like looking after a baby, we would give the body a bedtime routine to recognise; a warm bath, warm milky drink, curtains drawn as dusk arrived.

Auntie became aggressive at times. Once when I was assisting my dad at the leisure centre, she hit me in the face and then asked me what was I going to do about it? Everyone's eyes were upon me, clearly wondering how I was going to cope with this. I think people were always surprised by my calmness when they witnessed such events, but we had all realised that it was important to remember it wasn't really her but the illness. Although she had often revealed spoilt behaviour before the illness, she had never been aggressive. After that particular incident, I developed a huge bruise and she enquired with concern as to what had happened to me so I just gently told her a child had thrown a toy at me, by mistake.

When I went shopping with Auntie, I would have to observe her closely. If she saw an item, she fancied, she would pop it in my handbag! Fortunately, I always seemed to observe this because otherwise we could have ended up before the security team.

We tried to get household repairs performed by people who Auntie had already met because a stranger in the home was very unsettling for her but obviously this wasn't always possible. On one occasion we had a gentleman of colour helping Paul fit some kitchen units. Her description of the man which she shouted up to my dad was awful, but the extremely gracious worker laughed it off. As he left, he gave us a copy of the Bible – guess he thought we all needed the support living with Auntie.

On our final holiday abroad, before Dad had his heart attack, we thoroughly enjoyed Las Vegas. Paul and I returned to find my exhausted father, who felt bad about asking us to consider never leaving him again in charge of Auntie. He realised he couldn't cope after all; he had suffered from little sleep. Auntie had such energy as if she was fitted with Duracell batteries and she was very demanding. We came to accept the fact that we might never venture abroad again but it didn't really bother us if we could no longer travel, because we felt we had enjoyed our full quota of world sightseeing. I constantly thought to myself, 'I only get one Dad and I'm glad to be able to do all I can for him. 'So, no more bumping into Omar Sharif on a beach in Egypt, if only to exchange, 'Good Evening.'

After that, when we took Dad away for a one-week holiday each year, we placed Auntie in a residential home not too far away. It wouldn't have worked to have respite care in our own home because she'd have been so distressed if strangers were there instead of us. As I took Dad and Auntie everywhere with me, we didn't feel the need for day centres because we provided so much stimulation. In the care home, they had a pianist and when he played, Auntie would sit, happy and contented. However, the moment he stopped she would be trying to escape! When we went to drop her off, I would stay for a while to settle her in. When we observed some of the behaviour, we knew why we preferred to provide a home for Auntie with us. One lady kept coming into the lounge where another man was watching Wimbledon on the television. She asked him, 'Is this cricket or football?' and he explained it was tennis. The lady wandered out and, on her return, asked the same question. This happened three times until the man nearly lost it, 'You ask me that again and you'll get this chair over your head!' We learnt that it was best if Paul didn't accompany me to the care home, as there was a particular lady who was certain that Paul was an 'old flame' who had ditched her. She kept following him around shouting abuse at him, so I used to take Auntie in on my own in the end, far easier for all concerned!

Unfortunately, she hated the care home. We tried to speak to her daily on the phone but she couldn't work out where we were and it distressed her. She couldn't understand where she was and annoyed a male patient by going into his room, sitting on his toilet and then dressing in his clothes. Also, the staff informed us that she preferred his room to her own so didn't want to leave that room. She tried to escape by running down the garden and scaling the wall. Such distressed behaviour confirmed for us how important it was that we tried our utmost to keep Auntie in our family home despite her worsening condition. We couldn't bear the thought of her experiencing such confusion in unfamiliar surroundings without her family.

After our holiday we raced to pick her up. Auntie was sat happily chatting to a man and woman. As soon as she saw us, she said, 'I'm off!' The couple said, 'Well you said you'd got nobody!' Auntie just said, 'I can't help that.' And stood up to come with us. The man said to the other woman, 'She looks like a nice woman, let's see if we can go with her. Go and ask her if we can go too!'

I discovered that Auntie liked painting by numbers although as her condition grew worse, she couldn't concentrate sufficiently. During the last few months, she would just sit and stare at the walls where she would comment on the pink elephants that she could see dancing and we would pretend that we could too! Auntie Rita enjoyed going for car rides but it could become tedious for whoever was driving because she repeated the same question every few minutes, 'Do you enjoy driving?'

Dad enjoyed chess so we sorted out a computerised chess board for him, and we'd smile to ourselves as we heard him arguing with it, 'You can't do that, it's cheating!' Paul was very good with Dad and would take him for a round of golf followed by a bacon sandwich. Paul had a good father/son relationship with my dad and he learnt a lot from him.

Auntie was becoming more and more incontinent but adult nappies would be ripped off. It became a habit to pull her pants down and just go to the toilet wherever she was. I constantly had to watch her to look for signs that she might need the loo and I'd be asking her every few minutes if she'd come to the bathroom with me. We got so used to the stink of vomit and faeces that I used to joke we could serve it up as a side dish and we wouldn't have recoiled! I often arrived home at 2 a.m. from a night shift to discover faeces smeared all over the walls. There was nothing I could do but hold my breath while I set about cleaning and disinfecting. I built a cleaning stock which Mrs Hinch would have been envious of!

Sometimes Auntie would shock herself when looking in the mirror, just who was that old woman staring back? In her mind, Auntie was now back in her twenties! All our bedrooms had mirror sliding-door wardrobes which were really heavy but one day she pulled all the ones in her room over, smashing all the electrics. She told us all that Dad had done it. 'Do you think I'm crackers?' she'd say.

At birthdays or Christmas, I'd try to think of gifts that would make her happy and I would ask Dad if there were any special interests he could recall from her childhood. She enjoyed unwrapping her gifts and liked the pretty nail varnishes I had found for her in her favourite colours. For clothes, she liked beige, green and navy, no bright colours.

Pretty pyjamas and slippers appealed to her and small boxes of chocolate – she had a thing about not putting weight on. She liked to think she wasn't being greedy but in reality, she could wolf food down and often did, never putting weight on, lucky lady! She only weighed seven stone! I nearly died of embarrassment one day when we were leaving the leisure pool. I cringed the moment I noticed the obese lady we passed as I knew Auntie would comment and sure enough, she did: – 'Look at the backside on her! I don't know how she'll get round the gym!' Even though Auntie was a tiny lady, just four foot 11 inches, she preferred tall people.

To try and provide a bit of festive atmosphere we'd book to go to the various favourite pubs and restaurants for Christmas lunch and boxing day lunch.

We would always take her out for her birthday. My closest friends would often attend to provide a bit of a party group. Auntie would order a 12-ounce steak so I would pretend to pop to the loo but actually reorder a more fair-sized portion!

As the illness progressed, I continued to chat to Auntie even though it was so frustrating when she just stared into space. I sometimes thought I might as well have spoken a foreign language. Whatever I said the response would always be, 'Shall we go for a walk?' However, I would persevere and chat about simple things which wouldn't add to her confusion and general things which would relate to present and past times. The weather was a good topic because she was often mentally back in time!

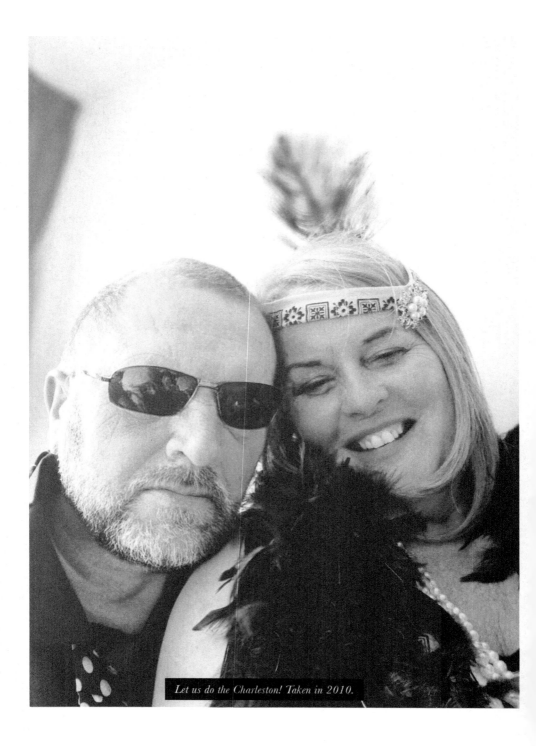

Let us do the Charleston! Taken in 2010.

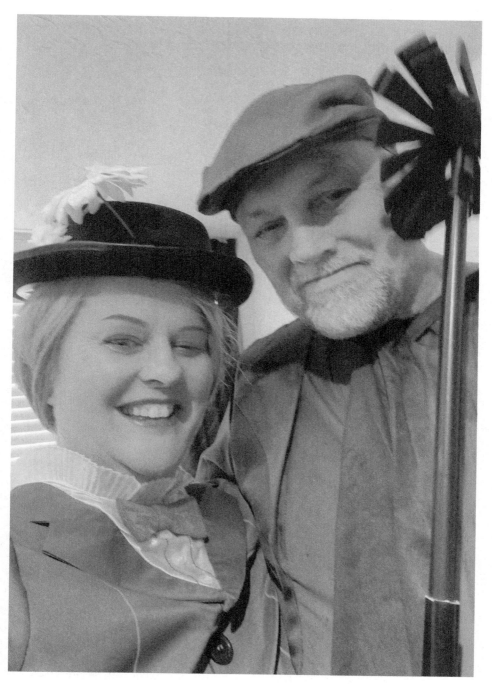

Have a waltz dressed as Mary Poppins and Bert in 2013.

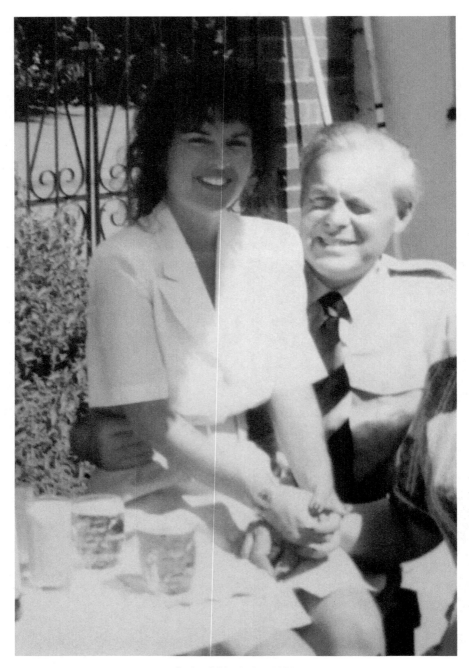

Dad and I in the late 1980s

4

HIDDEN ARMOUR – A SENSE OF HUMOUR

Things could get grim! We had to try and see the funny side of some of the more depressive episodes with Auntie. Laughter was so often our saviour.

We had decided to book a family holiday to the Isle of Wight. We soon realised we had taken a step too far when she tried to persuade the staff aboard the ferry that we had kidnapped her. This trick became a well-worn favourite with her! She was quite believable because physically she always looked perfect. I would always ensure that she was well dressed and her nails and hair were always done. She was smart and she had always kept herself trim all her life. She loved to wear jewellery and was very proud of some of her heirlooms. She always smelt lovely, washed with Imperial Leather soap. In fact, even nowadays in the house we get a waft of it! She had a bank of stock phrases that could be used in conversation, she could sound well educated and her story rang true so we had difficulty in assuring people that, in fact, she did have dementia.

The following vacation we felt it would be unkind to unsettle Auntie Rita by travelling so we researched the best local care homes which could offer respite care.

We continued to attend the leisure centre and one day as I sorted something for Dad, I asked a couple of the staff to keep an eye on Auntie. Distracted, they looked away for a few seconds – what a mistake! Auntie had done a runner. Because she always looked so presentable people always believed her little pleas for help, this time for a lift as she'd convinced her Good Samaritans that she had missed her bus. Leisure centre cameras saw her being whisked away! In desperation, I rang Paul who somehow managed to track her down as she was marching across the Merry Hill carparks. Another time Auntie decided to do a streak around the poolside. People reacted in such different ways, I guess it depended if they had any understanding of dementia. A businessman, there, was all for reporting the incident to the police, but another gentleman quickly grabbed a towel to wrap around Auntie and he patiently explained to the other man, not to be so silly, the lady had dementia. The problem was always highlighted because physically she looked well and was always beautifully presented. People felt affectionate and protective of her as she was a sweet, dainty, tiny lady.

At the spa, another day, she ran out of our car as we arrived and up to another couple and yet again complained that she had been kidnapped! Members of the public never ceased to amaze!

We had to involve the police on several occasions, and it would always help if they were handsome because then Auntie Rita would have no objections to being located by them if she had legged it whilst my attention was briefly diverted to the dogs. If they were ordinary looking, she would object profusely to going anywhere with them. On one occasion the police caught up with her and put handcuffs on her. The idea was to frighten her so that she wouldn't run off again but obviously that didn't sit very well with her. What she called the policemen can't really be repeated. As I keep stressing, she didn't look like she was ill and she could speak fluently, sometimes making what sounded like perfect sense.

Auntie should have been an Olympic sprinter, back in the day, because she became an expert as the disease progressed and could run away as if a mad bull was after her! Sometimes I resembled that mad bull in hot pursuit of her! She loved walking with me on Highgate Common and I asked if I could buy adult reins to prevent these mad dashes but apparently, it was against her human rights. One day dad needed my assistance, taking my eyes off her, away she ran! The warden and I frantically searched for her before having to resort yet again to calling the police. The carpark was closed as a precautionary measure. A constable on a bike and two officers in a patrol car searched for her only to find her sunbathing, flat on her back, enjoying the birdsong. It was the good-looking officer who found her and escorted her back. She was very fond of the older policemen as they seemed more in tune with her needs.

Looking back, I am surprised by how well the leisure centre tolerated us! On another occasion when we were in the pool area it was very quiet apart from another lady and her eight-year-old daughter who was learning to swim. Auntie was chattering away and appearing to make complete sense. The woman went out to change, leaving her daughter in the pool. I popped to the toilet. The woman smiled at me and said how nice it was to be able to leave her daughter in the capable hands of that champion swimmer! Auntie Rita couldn't even swim, but she certainly knew how to come up with a few tales! When I explained that Auntie had dementia and couldn't even swim the woman was naturally aghast!

The hairdressers would oblige by locking the door when Auntie was in the salon. One time I returned to collect her and to pay and discovered that Auntie was very angry. She ordered me not to pay the hairdresser because she claimed she'd dyed her hair the wrong colour. The poor girl was clearly mortified but I played along saying, yes it was dreadful, and we wouldn't pay. I winked at the girl who was desperately showing me the colour card with Auntie's choice. I managed to leave the money with a generous tip as I hurried Auntie away from the other, horrified, customers.

We had similar embarrassments at the dentists when she was fitted with her false teeth. That became another chore for me, bodyguard of those dentures, saving them from all sorts of accidents when Auntie decided to take them out and do goodness knows what with them.

We had been to Bridgnorth for a meal when Auntie Rita spotted a posh dress shop. She insisted on going in and immediately spotted a coat that took her fancy. On it went and her comments were broadcast for all to hear, 'It's a lovely colour but I think it makes me look a bit common. People might think I'm a bit of a tart in this, what do you think?'

'Excuse me that's my coat!' another customer demanded it back!

The medication for her heart eventually led to thinning of what had been a beautiful head of hair, so we got her some lovely wigs as Auntie's appearance had always been important to her. Numerous times we saw people giggle as she lifted the wig to scratch her head and then pop it back down, rather crooked! Jasper Carrott as Mr Wiggy watch out!

Some days were even harder than others. On one occasion when I turned to the doctor for help, he told me to drink red wine – that it was better than medication! I must admit our dogs and wine were the only things that made life seem fine on some days!

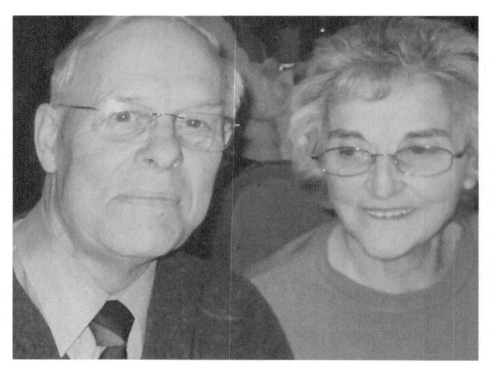

Dad and Auntie Rita at a birthday party circa 2010.

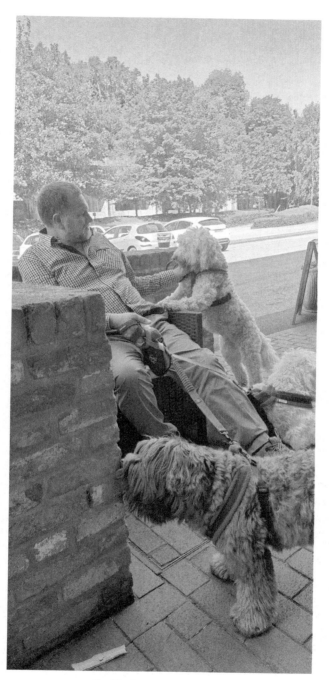

Paul having a chat with Rosie.

5

OH WHAT POSSIBILITIES!

So many people asked if we missed our previous existence, the ski trips, the romantic dinners for two, the opportunities to jet off to exotic holiday locations at a moment's notice. They seemed to dream up so many possibilities of things that had never even crossed our minds, but we always had the same answer: No, we had no regrets although there were moments where we felt like slitting our wrists!

Auntie suffered from sundowning, which usually started at dinnertime and continued into the night. Time meant nothing to her. She was topsy turvy and would think nothing of getting up at two in the morning to go a walk and then deciding to go to bed mid-morning. During this stage, she would display increased agitation, restlessness, irritability and confusion. We had to find ways to manage sundowning. We tried to use distraction techniques; sometimes it worked, sometimes it didn't. She might accept a drink or a snack. We'd try to offer physical comfort, but she didn't really like to be hugged or to hold hands. We experimented with diets and observed if certain foods had effects. Sometimes I thought Paul got off lightly because, as he arrived, everything was already done and Auntie Rita was about to go to bed, although that didn't mean that we had uninterrupted nights! Auntie could be all over the show in the night. I became a light sleeper as parents of young babies are and my antennae were programmed to wake me at the slightest noise! Dad was accustomed to his sister waking him at three in the morning for a hike which of course was not good for his heart condition! Often one of us would have to read to her in order to convince her to get back into bed and try to sleep. We got the Audible app for her in the end, hoping the soothing voice would calm her.

I could still listen to the music I loved or hypnotherapy by the marvellous Paul McKenna. I could still exercise and swim regularly. We had loved long-distance walking and we were lucky that Rita and Dad loved walking but of course, we had to scale down our lovely long hikes to much shorter routes. I was with my family and dogs, what more could I want – apart from more time! Some days there was barely time to bathe. Without a thought Paul and I were consistent in our convictions, 'We'd do it all again.'

We tried to involve Dad and Auntie in all our decisions and plans. Dad had chosen our dog, Bertie's, name. He liked watching Jeeves and Bertie Wooster. It was a Victorian name really and I felt floral names fitted in well – hence the choice of names for our other dogs. Bertie was especially close to my dad. Bertie was on permanent guard dog duty and allowed no outsider near my dad. He would carefully observe if anybody shook Dad's hand.

We were often very exhausted mentally and physically! It was quite common for Auntie Rita to arrive in our bed at any ungodly hour, clambering over us. If we were sat having a cuddle in the lounge and I was sat on Paul's knee she would climb on his other! Just as Princess Diana had complained I could easily moan, 'There's three of us in this marriage!' Any spare moments to be romantic, we grabbed them. Even at our silver wedding party, I had to sit at one table with Auntie Rita, Dad and friends while Paul sat at another with more guests.

Auntie's needs were the top priority, more so than Dad's because obviously her condition was more demanding. As the years went on, I realised how much I had sacrificed in some ways; for example I used to love wearing make-up and I'd try all the latest products. I would have all the 'war paint' on. Whereas I might once have Chanel No. 5 on my present wish list, it transformed into Dettol No. 5! Whereas I might have a cupboard full of make-up and be familiar with all the latest products I coveted a cupboard full of cleaning products! I am sure I could write a book that Cleaning Queens, Kim and Aggie, would long to read!

Cooking has always been a hobby of mine and I managed to carry on with this because Auntie Rita would sit and watch me. She was quite safe because she had no desire to join in, it had never been an interest of hers. However, due to the special diets I needed to adhere to for Dad and Auntie Rita, I couldn't experiment anymore with exotic dishes or anything a little bit different or special.

I did miss my friends; many couldn't cope with the fact that if they came round or if I went there, I had to be accompanied by Auntie Rita. Many couldn't find the empathy but I respected that if they had not experienced caring for a loved one with dementia that they might find it impossible to comprehend. Conversations were limited as Auntie would join in with nonsense or rudeness. Having never been racist, sexist or quite so openly outspoken before her illness, we could never be sure what unacceptable comments might pop out of her lips now, at the most embarrassing moments. We eventually stopped the dinner parties which we used to love hosting, pre-Auntie Rita days. Our final dinner party was the one where Auntie Rita came downstairs in her nightie. She sat herself at the table with us all and announced that the dog had cooked the meal. One of our guests remarked, 'But he's a dog!' Auntie Rita agitatedly responded, 'Do you think I'm an idiot? Of course he's a dog.' She insisted that he cooked fantastic food and did it every day. We eventually persuaded Auntie Rita to return to her room and our guest couldn't stop himself from commenting 'She's barking mad.' That's when we decided it wasn't fair to Auntie or our guests to have occasions like this. I actually made a friend because of Auntie Rita, in a way. Walking on Highgate Common, the lady often noticed Auntie dart behind a tree, and my new friend often joined us on our walks after that.

Auntie Rita used to hide food everywhere. She must have been quite clever because we usually kept her in our sight but even months after we had sadly lost her, we would say, 'Auntie Rita strikes again,' when we found some food which she'd stashed away in the most unexpected hiding place! She was quite ingenious really!

We never had time to feel lonely and after all, we had each other and our myriad of pets which Dad and Auntie loved; tortoises, cats and of course our precious dogs. Auntie Rita would do anything to entice the cats to snuggle up in her bed.

As a child, we had a household of cats, and I loved our blue Persian cat who I would stroke from top to tail before Mum had pointed out to me that I was annoying the cat. I understood when Mum demonstrated by brushing my hair just as roughly. We didn't get a dog until I was ten when I was given an apricot poodle, called Tango, for my birthday but he wasn't interested in me! He would growl whenever he saw me and he only wanted my mum! Mind you, I did used to play hide the butcher's bone with him, which didn't exactly endear him to me!! I just thought it was fun – now I realise that I was teasing him!

It was because of Auntie that we had added to our dog family. She really liked the idea of a new dog and at that time I was fancying a rottweiler, so we travelled to Blackpool where I had seen some advertised by the Kennel Club. A lovely lady welcomed us into her home to view the puppies. Now, Auntie just took herself off upstairs, we assumed to 'powder her nose', the owner of the dogs just watched her, I think a bit taken aback; we explained that she had dementia and apologised. Then we heard her pull the chain, we seemed to have been fussing over the puppies for ages and we were conscious of the lady glancing up the stairs as I began to wonder just where Auntie had got to? I worried that she might have done what had become a recent habit – stripping off. I asked if I could just pop up to check she was ok. I nervously wondered what we were going to encounter. There lay Auntie Rita, curled up, in the lady's bed, with her husband, perhaps he had woken and thought he was dreaming. Auntie Rita went on to say she didn't like rottweilers and she wanted a 'teddy bear dog.' This comment led us to our love of labradoodles. The three other dogs, we have since bought, have been the making of Bertie, he loves his little harem!

Paul's father had tragically committed suicide a year after our marriage. Suffering from PTSD (Post-traumatic stress disorder) from the war, he had struggled mentally for years. We had gone to Cornwall with my parents and grandmother. When we arrived home from vacation Paul found a note pushed through our door asking him to phone his mum. What a shock to hear Paul's dad, who couldn't swim, had thrown himself into the local canal. It was a tragic moment for everyone.

On one of our earlier family meals, we had all ordered our desserts. Auntie Rita eyed them all up as they arrived, and she immediately made the decision that she was having the biggest, most scrumptious looking pudding even though my sister-in-law had ordered it and was now left with Auntie's boring-looking plain tiny effort. Auntie always enjoyed all the getting ready, the manicures, the hairdressing – I eventually went down the mobile hairdresser route. She adored wearing a new posh frock. However, once this getting ready session was over, she would play up terribly when it came time to actually go to the restaurants with friends and family.

I enjoyed reflexology. Auntie Rita would settle down for her session after flicking through her favourite Hello magazine, attracted by the colourful photographs. I had developed a sensitive stomach, mainly after my mother passed away, but reflexology helped incredibly.

We have a holiday home in Wales, and we felt lucky and grateful that we could still take breaks here. Auntie Rita did put us under a few stresses there, however. For example, one day Paul and I were on the decking while Dad was having a wash in the bathroom. We heard distressed shouts when he returned to his bedroom to discover he had no clothes left because Auntie Rita had thrown them all out of the window. Maybe she thought the glass was the door

THE DOG ALWAYS COOKS

to a washing machine and that she was being helpful! Her response to our question, 'Why did you do that?' was always guaranteed to be the same – that it wasn't her who'd done it! We always tried to make the most out of the time that we all had together. The one time at one of our holiday homes, it was the 80th birthday of Dad. Now, we had kept telling him that a celebrity was flying in for his birthday celebrations. We said we had paid a considerable amount of money for this to happen. It couldn't have been timed any better, when Paul left the room to change him and put a Mr. Bean mask on, a helicopter flew overhead and landed in the next field (don't know why).

Dad's face was a picture, initially, for the first minute or so when Paul re-entered the room.

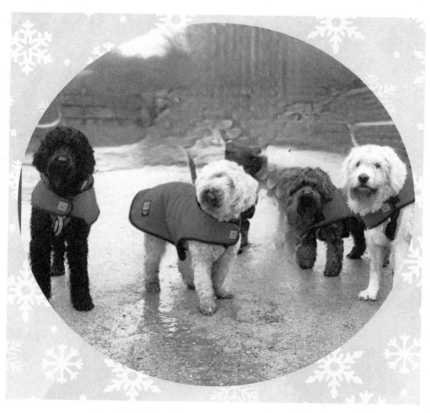

From left to right: Lily, Rosie, Daisy and Bertie in 2021.

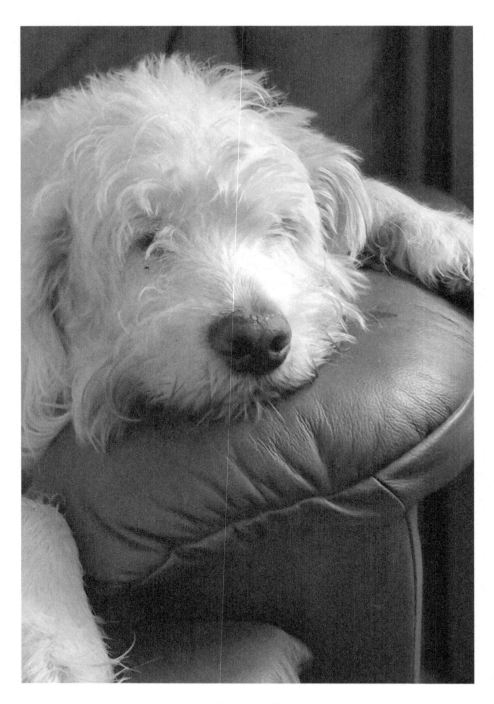

Bertie, the dancing doodle in 2021.

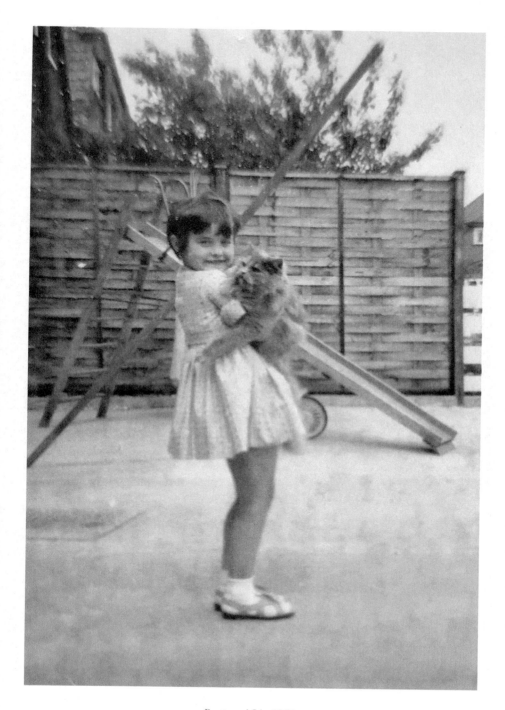

Bunty and I in 1968.

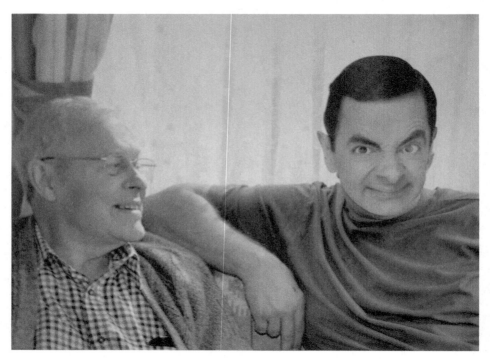

Dad and 'Mr. Bean' at our holiday home in Builth Wells.

6

THANK YOU FOR THE MUSIC

Paul and I met in a nightclub. He reckons that he'd already had his eye on me! He jumped in at his chance to be my knight in shining armour when I dropped my purse, and my coins went everywhere! Eighteen months later we were engaged, and a year after that we married on 21 July 1984, five days before my birthday. Paul had asked my dad for my hand before he took me on holiday to Wales. He had insisted that day that we went walking up the Great Orme to show me something! Upon reaching the summit, whilst I was taking in the spectacular scenery, Paul went to get a bottle of water out of his rucksack; he then got down on one knee and presented me with this beautiful engagement ring. Whilst this was going on a few people had appeared and they started clapping. Upon getting back up his seam split in his trousers, which caused much amusement to all. Made no difference though, he still produced a bottle of Bollinger and two champagne flutes from his rucksack. Dad always joked it was the excitement of the situation! I had a glorious wedding with four bridesmaids and a page boy. We enjoyed our honeymoon in Cornwall.

I soon realised what a good husband I had in Paul; he took everything in his stride. So many people have pointed out that we must have had a very strong relationship to survive such constant intrusion. Paul had willingly adapted our house to accommodate Dad and his sister and he had made a huge loft conversion for us so that Dad and Auntie Rita could have adjoining bedrooms on the same floor. Paul always showed nothing but consideration for the comfort of our two new family members and we even converted the garage into an additional bedsit as Auntie's dementia progressed. We were aware that stairs might become an issue for her safety. The growing demands and needs of both our relatives magnified further what a steadfast relationship Paul and I had. We had both agreed to always place Dad and Aunties' needs as a top priority and to accept that, in the pecking order of things, we were at the bottom!

Paul was amazing with my dad and auntie. I don't know any other man who would ask for special shifts at work for no other reason than they could come home and care for two elderly people, fitting in with my work schedule. They weren't even blood-related to him but Paul grew to love Dad, especially, and was always fond of Auntie.

He told me recently how, when I was out, he'd defy my strict healthy diet and treat Dad to a chocolate or two! Apparently, when he took Dad for a haircut, he'd treat him to a bacon sandwich – Dad was always delighted!

Paul used to say going to work was a relief in the end and he felt sorry for me because I got no relief. He said he enjoyed the banter at work. He had some hilarious moments. One day his bank made a flash mistake. For a brief, few minutes £1,000,000 popped into his account. Paul got a quick camera shot of his affluent bank account before the bank rectified things. So, Paul thought to himself, 'I'm going to have fun with this!' He waited until everyone had gone and then he said to his friend, 'Can I let you in on a secret? I don't want you to tell anybody.'

At first, his mate wouldn't believe Paul's claim that he had become a millionaire but once he showed him, on his phone, the friend was gobsmacked! 'You're very cool about it. Will you leave your job?' Paul explained that he felt he owed the company which had been good to him, so he'd complete the week. Once Paul starts a joke, he can take it a step too far. He's a bit of a devil for stringing it out! Paul went out to his car and then came back and announced he would leave there and then actually and would his friend like a job as a chauffeur for me! The friend's eyes nearly popped out of his head at Paul's offer of a starting salary of £50,000! He even started to write his resignation letter! Finally, Paul thought he better tell his friend the truth, 'I'm having you on.' But his mate took much convincing!

Paul and I share a great sense of humour and it's one of the main things that carried us through the difficult moments, not forgetting the dogs and the wine! Paul always had a wonderful time on April Fool's Day and often tried to include me in his pranks! His manager had never met me before so when he saw Paul with me for the first time, he asked, 'Who's this?' so Paul told him I was his girlfriend and not to tell anybody! The boss, of course, did tell everyone as he went for a snack in the canteen but when the others got him to describe me, they said, 'He's having you on. That's his wife!' When he worked at the buses and there were a few problems with some of the services he made me ring his colleague pretending to be the local Press, wanting to run a feature on the absent bus service. Paul was in hysterics as his colleague told me to wait while he went to get his manager because he was the only person there in reality! When Paul (my editor) went on the line to speak to him, he gave Paul a few choice words. He did see the joke ... eventually! Paul always alleviated his stress with a good laugh. He's a proper wind-up merchant, my husband!

Paul kept me sane, and I couldn't have faced the journey I took without him beside me. It would have been so lonely without my amazing hubby!

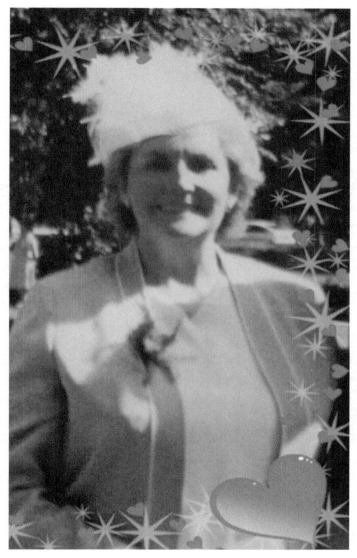

My mum on our wedding day.

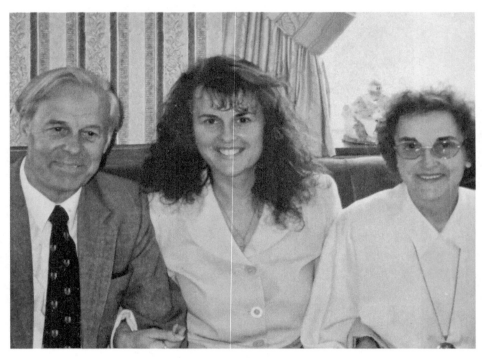

Dad, Auntie Rita and I at Terrace restaurant, Cannock in the 1990s.

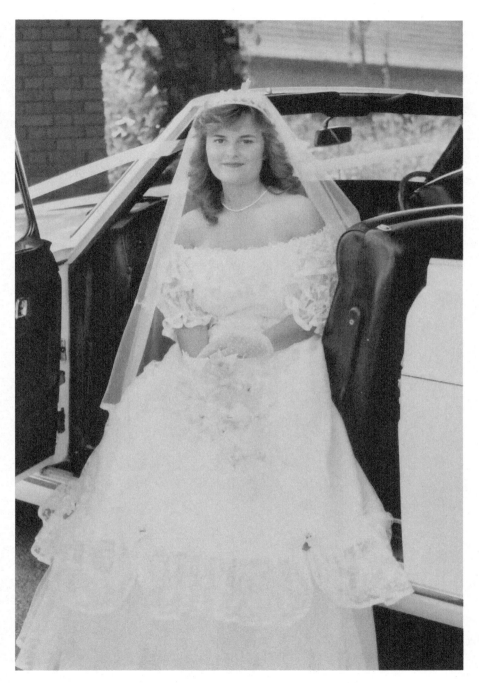

My glorious wedding day in 1984.

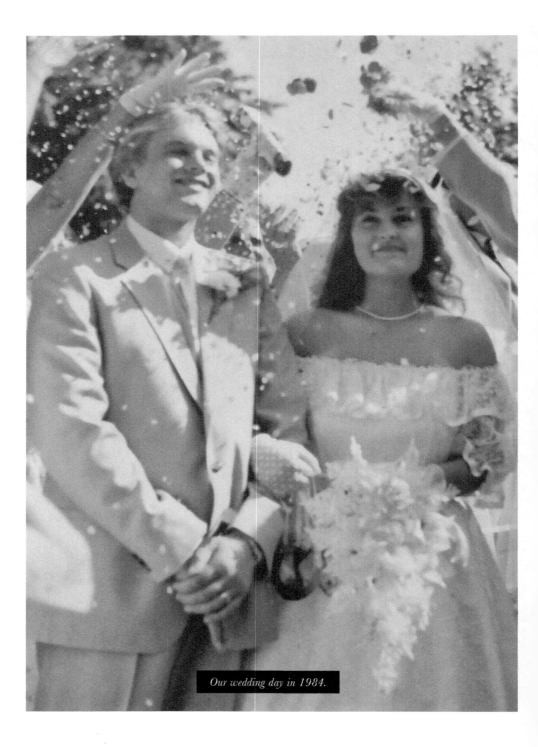

Our wedding day in 1984.

7

OFF TO WORK WE GO!

I enjoyed my job in the ambulance service because a vocation where I could help others was always my ambition. I had always wanted to be a policewoman and my application took me to Lloyd House in Birmingham where unfortunately it ended because of my height! In those days, women had to be five foot six and I wasn't, so the recruiting officer said, 'If you grow little one, come back!'

I had to keep dropping my hours at work. The ambulance service was amazing, so supportive. In the end, I was just working eight hours – four on the Monday and four on a Friday. They even let me change roles, so I was just working in dispatch in the end. Paul worked in the head office at National Express and they also showed compassion and support by allowing Paul to work the shifts that fitted in with my job. Therefore, there was always one of us at home to supervise Auntie Rita and to nurse Dad.

I am not sure if many completely understood the stress I

71

was under, although they would have noticed the evolution from, 'relaxed woman,' to 'fairly uptight woman!' One of the calls that I had taken at work, turned out to be a murder case and, unfortunately, it had been expected that I'd attend the court sessions so my doctor had to explain that this was not possible due to my commitment with Auntie.

Keeping calm was one of the most important things in my job. Any hint of panic in my voice would have had terrible knock-on consequences for the person on the other end of the phone. In addition, I had to learn to control my emotions. For example, my tears wanted to fall when an old lady rang, on the return from her shopping trip, to say she had discovered that her husband had hung himself. I had to glide through each call like a swan and keep the person talking, in some cases, until the crew could get to them. I often felt a gut reaction when taking calls as to the severity of the situation. There was often an increase in false calls during the school holidays. On one occasion a child rang claiming he'd just run out to the shop for some crisps and pop, and he'd seen an accident. He said the ambulance would spot himself as he had red hair and a red jumper. It all sounded so suspect that I thought, 'I bet you have!' in my head but my professional voice reassured the kid that we would be on our way. It turned out there actually was a little kid with red hair in a red jumper waiting to flag down the ambulance!

We had all sorts of calls including one from a burglar,

with a conscience, who just shouted, 'Ambulance,' down the phone before scarpering. The paramedics found an old man who'd fallen down the stairs as he had chased the intruders. I admired the pregnant lady and her four-year-old son as she rang from the bath, in labour. The four-year-old had to climb on a stool to open the door to our team as she shouted directions to her son. She'd got into the bath to prevent all the mess from ruining her carpets!

Finishing work on the two a.m. shifts was always difficult and to be honest, at times scary! After one such shift, I approached my car, in deep snow, to meet a man dragging a huge suitcase across the car park. Having recently watched too many crimes programmes my brain told me there was a body in that suitcase! 'Did I make you jump? Have you got the time, love?' the weird looking man asked as I scurried into my car and locked the door.

After another 2 a.m. finish, as I was driving home, I observed a woman lying on the carriageway. Bear in mind, I was not really sure if it was genuine, or some kind of hoax. I had seen situations on the television where drivers had pulled over to help and been 'carjacked'. So, I decided to pull over when I could, and phone into the control room. I had a huge stuffed gorilla, so I started to keep him in my car, in the passenger seat, wearing a cap and scarf. In the dark, it would appear as if I was accompanied by a hulk of a male! When Auntie saw gorilla-man in my car, she never batted an eyelid! She actually wanted to know where I had met him. My uniform colours changed from navy to green and if Auntie heard me when I returned from these late-night shifts, she'd ask if I was returning from school or sometimes, she thought I worked for the council and that I was returning from a gardening session. I'd always play along with what she was saying. Dad was always proud of me in my role and carried a photograph of me in my uniform, everywhere he went. Auntie Rita showed no interest, she really didn't understand where I went each day!

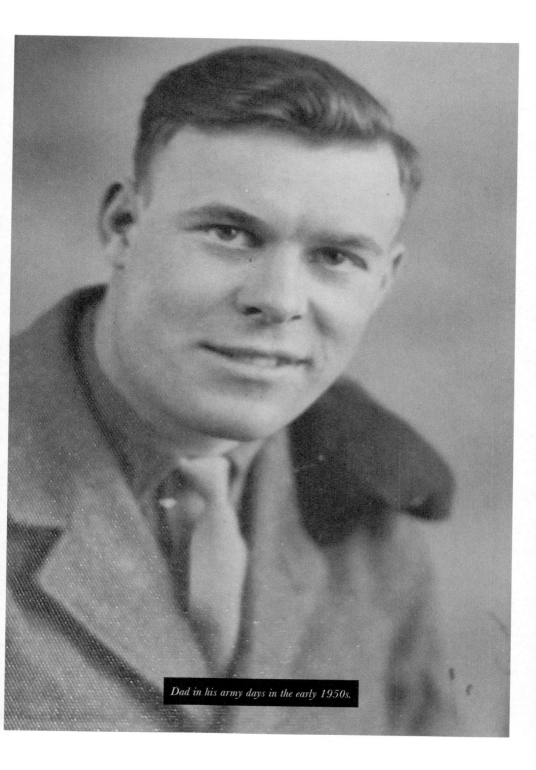

Dad in his army days in the early 1950s.

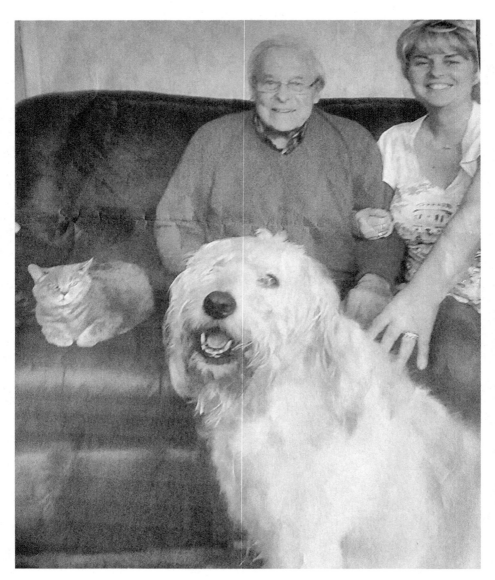

Dad, Bertie, Elsa and I.

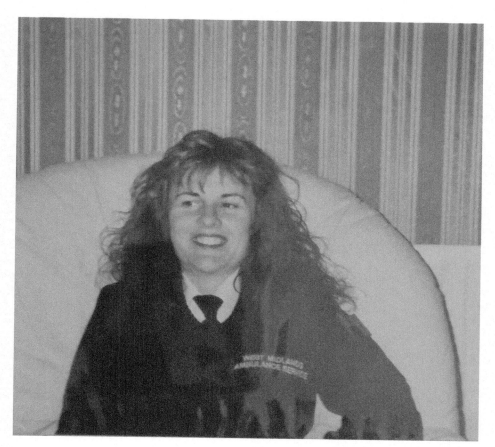

Me ready to go to work in 1995

8

TIPS TO HELP OTHERS ADAPT TO A SIMILAR CARING ROLE

E very case of dementia is different, and every patient has their own individual needs but I thought a few tips might help any reader who is considering the journey of home care for a loved one with dementia.

1. Sew labels in your loved one's clothes marked with their name and address. Unfortunately, the disease can cause wandering or the desire to return to their childhood home or to a favourite place from the past.
2. Put room names on each door so the patient can find their way around.
3. Make sure you have good window and door locks and place the keys where you can find them in an emergency.
4. Hide any precious jewellery because bright things attract, and they could get thrown down the toilet!

5. Ask for the medical teams to come to you e.g., with flu injections, as dementia patients can find it very distressing to be taken out of their daily routine.

6. Buy bed guards, over the bed trays plus mattress protectors, beaker mugs and dementia cutlery.

7. If the patient doesn't appear to be speaking sense try to interpret their wishes by observing their body language.

8. Don't offer complex choices, keep things basic and use short sentences, trying to make eye contact with the patient.

9. Be aware that rugs can be tripping hazard and that food temperatures need to be checked. The dementia mind will not register that something like soup is too hot to eat.

10. Lay out clothes in the order they'll be put on and be prepared to dress the patient. If the patient wears incontinence pads and repeatedly tries to remove them try buying onesies.

11. Wet wipes are invaluable, always carry some in your handbag.

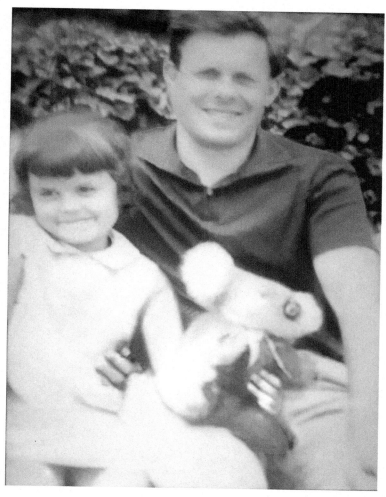

Dad, Me and Koala!

9

OUR JOURNEY FORWARD BEGAN WITH SMALL STEPS

Love is rare, we grabbed it when it came our way and gave it from every pore of our hearts. We are learning to live with our grief and Dad and Auntie Rita are captured in our memories forever. They make us smile as we face whatever is going on in our present lives.

'Stone the crows,' Auntie used to say, a catchphrase of hers. How we missed that voice of hers when she left us. How I missed Dad's easy-going ways and his peaceful presence, my wonderful father!

We were lucky that they both passed in their sleep. It was terrible snowy weather when Auntie Rita died, and the undertakers could not get to collect her for two days so it was incredibly distressing. Usually, either Paul or I would check on Dad and Auntie Rita at about half eleven each night. However, sadly on 18th December 2010 when we went into Auntie Rita's bedroom, we found that she had passed away. This left us in a huge shock. Paul has no belief in ghosts so he was absolutely shocked when he saw her going to the kitchen after her death. All three of us had this identical experience on completely different occasions. We interpreted it to mean that she hadn't yet realised that she had passed, or maybe it was because we weren't ready to let go of her.

How my heart broke again when we lost Dad last February, aged ninety years and six months. Apparently, he had prostate cancer, but he died from his heart problems. The doctors had predicted that he would live for six years after his heart attack but we were blessed that he lived for fourteen years. I like to think that we contributed to this because of the round the clock care he was given. We had lost Auntie Rita seven years previously and I found her funeral service so upsetting. Obviously, there were few mourners to attend and support us. Dad had chosen, 'Time to Say Goodbye,' by Katherine Jenkins to play at his sister's funeral. It was heart-wrenching. With Dad, we decided not to have a funeral. The undertakers removed his body from our home. We found it heart-warming to receive his ashes back, delivered to us in a beautiful urn. I don't think I could have attended a funeral, due to my grief. I had found Auntie's funeral devastating. I am going to have a beautiful necklace or bracelet crafted which will contain some of Dad's ashes and Paul is going to have a ring containing ashes.

Dad particularly loved walking on Highgate Common so we go there often to sit on the bench we erected in his memory. It bears the words, 'Let this bench bring peace to all who sit on it.' I like to think there is an afterlife. If I see a robin, when I'm sat on Dad's bench, I believe in the saying that when a robin is here, a loved one is near. Auntie Rita had requested to be buried so she lies in a grave in Dudley church with a simple headstone and we visit regularly.

We keep ourselves busy decorating. Paul is refurbishing the whole house, but we see memories of our two lost loved ones everywhere. We are gradually making our house less clinical.

The dogs keep us busy and we haven't ruled out adding a red one to our pack from the same breeder. We have been to training classes with some of them. Bertie is the only dog and he got as far as his silver medal but because we had never had him neutered, he could go no further. At the end of the day, hormones will overbalance any amount of training! If a bitch in season tempts Bertie, he'll go despite how many Barbara Woodhouse inspired trainers shout after him! I walk miles with them; I can easily cover twelve miles because I sometimes walk them in pairs due to their differing needs. Bertie is old and doesn't need to go so far. The dogs need so much attention that it's almost like the old days of being full-time carers. I just bought lots of ball launchers so that they are distracted on walks and don't tease each other! All the coping skills I developed to help with Auntie are coming in handy with these mischievous imps. They egg each other on! Just as I did with Auntie and Dad, I spoil them rotten and I just couldn't resist buying them a pig's trotter each, today, when I was buying mince to make beef burgers for training treats for them.

Paul won't travel abroad without the dogs but encourages me to go on holiday with a friend if I want. However, we are content holidaying in this country where we can take our four dogs. I also have Suzy, a very beautiful chestnut horse. I have always enjoyed riding but about twenty-five years ago I put two back discs out. Before then I had gained my brown belt in karate.

Caring for our pets is so therapeutic and animals have always brought us so many blessings. We had three tortoises for over twenty-five years. When Auntie and Dad were with us, I decided there was one area we could make life easier. I discovered a vet, down South, who would be happy to take our tortoises. She grew all her own produce so I knew they'd be well cared for. I didn't really think I loved the tortoises, there's not really a way you can have a relationship with them, but we did our best by them!

I love caring for the elderly so I might do some voluntary work in the future… maybe! Paul and I have developed so many new skills through our experiences. However, I have never been one for planning for the future and just live from day to day. My sister-in-law suggested a plan that when she retires, we could start up a dog walking business together, sounds like a good idea.

We are still recovering, and I enjoy acupuncture to help

me relax. We also have a hot tub and sauna where we relax most evenings with a glass of red wine ... naturally!

We have our own house rental business which keeps us very busy because Paul does all the renovations. He also renovates properties as a favour for his friends. We just don't have enough hours in the day for all the things we do right now. We do favours for people when we can. This week we looked after a friend's two Labradors for him so you can imagine it was rather hectic here with six dogs running around!

My memories are still very raw. I am studying for a degree in health and social care with the Open University which is helping me to come to terms with the events of recent years.

Dad passed away a month before lockdown commenced but it felt no different to us as we had been in lockdown for fourteen years. Dad had always reminded me during the tough times that there was always somebody worse off and I hope this book helps others to find their positives as they journey along.

I'd do it all again in a heartbeat. We have no regrets, everything led us to the place we are now where we hope our experiences can help others.

I hope you have enjoyed this book, I have tried to make a terribly sad situation as light-hearted as possible.

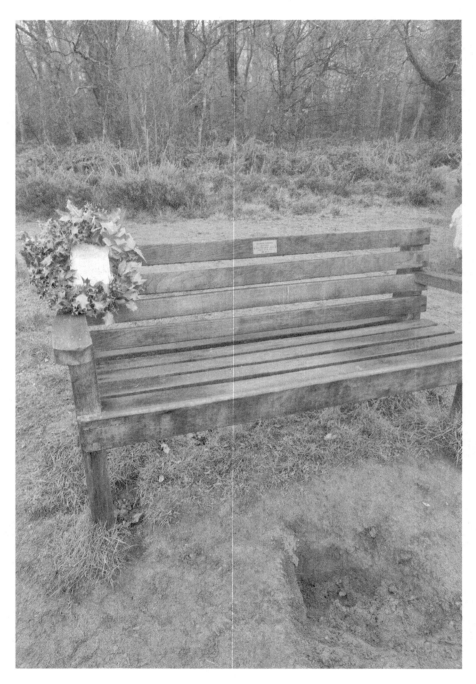

Memorial bench for Dad on Highgate Common, 2021.

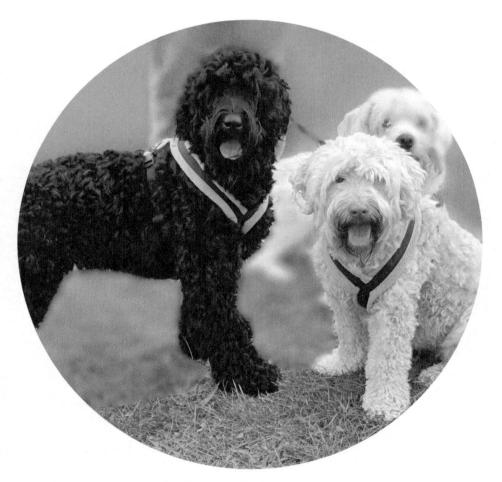

Our lovely dogs: Lily, Rosie and Bertie.

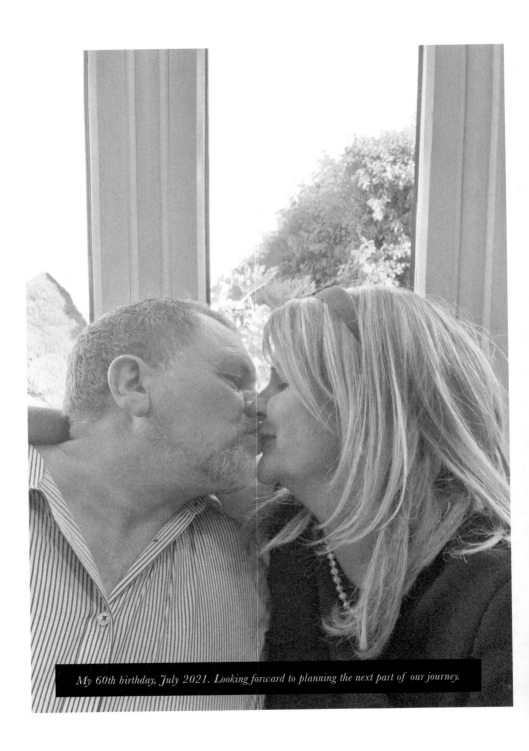

My 60th birthday, July 2021. Looking forward to planning the next part of our journey.

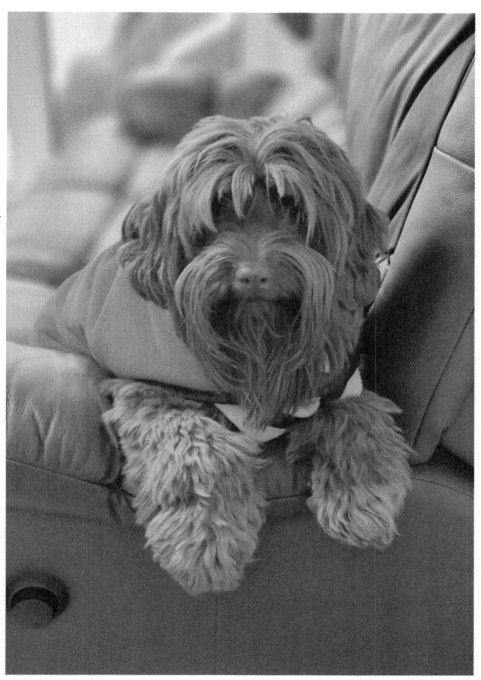

Daisy, one of our beautiful dogs.

StoryTerrace

Printed in Great Britain
by Amazon

11639431R00054